# The Patient's Guide to Pain Management

(Become a Pain Warrior)

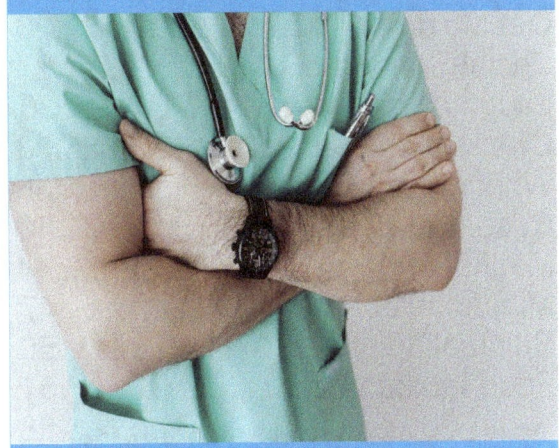

Real World Solutions
Regain Your Life

MATTHEW DOVIE MS, PA-C

# Table of Contents

# Introduction

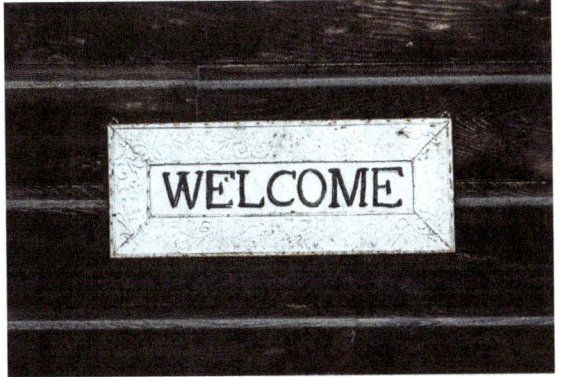

Welcome and congratulations as you have taken the first step to becoming an active participant in finding an effective treatment for your pain.

Success in the world of managing chronic and acute pain is relative to the individual. My hope for you is to improve your quality of life and give you insightful information to become the owner of your condition.

I will provide information and advice in a 4 staged multidisciplinary approach to help you find success in topics ranging from Health, Wellness, Traditional Medicine and Lifestyle Modifications.

I have spent the last 23 years in practice designing this Patient's Guide to Pain Management. My goal is to empower you and motivate you to live your best life.

We will begin with an overview and then dive into concrete medical treatments.

# Active Participant

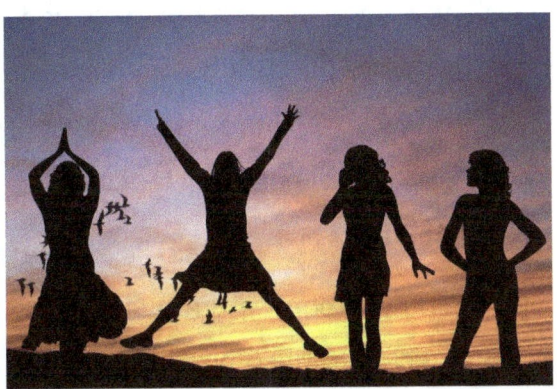

It is important for all patients to be involved as an active participant in their treatment plan. This seems obvious but too many patients take a passive approach to their healing and care.

Too many times I have treated patients who don't follow the recommendations and plans given to them and then are surprised when they haven't made any progress. As you know, treating pain is complex. You must treat both the physical, emotional, psychological and spiritual nature of one's being to find long term benefit. There are no shortcuts and no magic pill that will take all the pain away.

By reading this book you are taking a good first step to becoming an active participant in your care. My goal is to show you ways to become further involved as an active participant including nutrition, exercise, meditation, medication and exciting interventional pain treatments.

I'm excited you have decided to join me on this journey.

# Be a Champion!

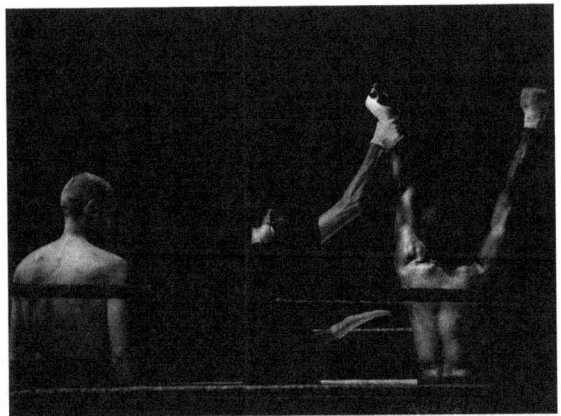

To effectively treat your pain you must learn to become a champion. A champion is defined as an individual who overcomes great odds to achieve their goals.

This is an active approach to taking back your life. The first step is to pick one activity that you had quit due to you pain. This can be as simple as walking up the hill to the mailbox or going to the grocery store. There is no quit in a champion, you will start by telling your pain "I'm taking this back!". As you start to slowly add back more activities you will gain more confidence and improve your quality of life. These small victories will improve your mood and outlook. Just like any champion, the road to success will have its highs and lows. Don't become frustrated if you have a setback, only by failing can we learn to succeed.

By winning more and more of these small victories you will learn to control your pain and not let your pain control you. When you learn that you control your pain you will become a champion!

# Find your team!

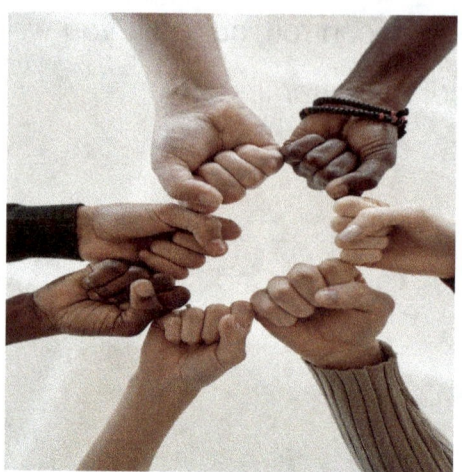

To treat your pain you will need to actively seek a health care team dedicated to achieving your goals. I hope to weaponize you with actionable information to help you begin this journey. You will want to seek providers that take a multidimensional approach. Ideally you will have a healthcare provider who can help you manage any issues needed. Find a provider that doesn't treat you like cattle. Find a provider that takes the time to know their patients and not someone who kicks you out the door after 10 minutes. Avoid the 'pill mill' clinics! If you suffer with underlying anxiety and depression, which is almost every patient, you will want to also work with a pain psychologist or psychiatrist to help with coping skills.

Some additional treatments that I recommend would involve joining a a pain support group, either one specifically for your pain condition or one for chronic pain. Having a support group to vent at, share ideas, share victories or frustrations is a critical component to healing.

I like to call it the "Oprah effect" as Oprah has done wonders with addressing issues and bringing them into the viewer's living room. So can these support groups be your "Oprah effect".

As you become a more active participant, I then encourage my patients to actively seek an exercise instructor with experience in pain patients. Yoga, Tai Chi, Pilates, aquatic therapy are all wonderful examples of improving strength and flexibility while decreasing pain.

The goal is finding the right members to fill out your pain fighting team!

## Learn Patience

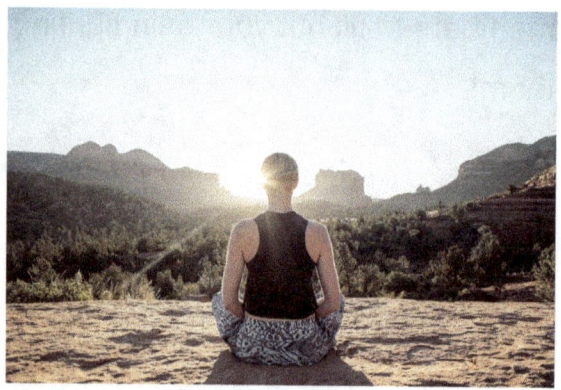

To treat your pain a patient must learn patience. Your chronic pain is a complex web that developed through a course of unfortunate events and set up an ingrained neurological pathway signal of pain to your brain. I give the example of a girl walking across a dewy meadow. A girl walks across the meadow in the morning, you would not see her path later in the day. However, if that same girl walks across the meadow everyday for the next 6 months, even if she then misses one day you will be able to see the path she has walked. This is the same as chronic pain patterns.

It took a long time to get to the point of your chronic pain and your treatment will also take a period of time and be a process to heal.

Don't expect any magical healthcare provider to be able to solve all your problems in one visit.

Instead, understand that a patient with patience and understanding will have the best results. Patience also helps to curb anxiety that intensifies pain and hinders the healing process.

I recommend mindful meditation, prayer, exercise or relaxation techniques to help patients practice patience. These techniques will help decrease stress cortisol levels, boost natural endorphins and will help patients become more in tune with their body and help the healing process.

# Be Proactive

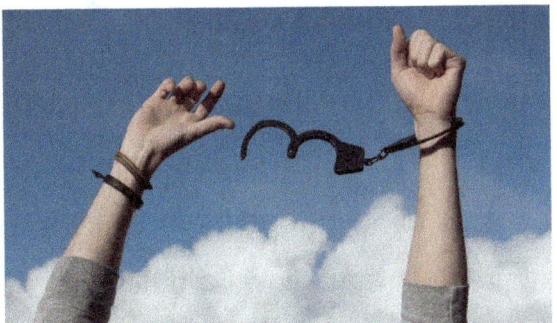

Although this was stated above, it is
worth repeating and describing
further.  To help find an effective
treatment for you pain, I require my
patients to become proactive. This
requires patients to take the
initiative to improve their situation.
Instead of letting your current
circumstances be the driving force
of determining your future I help
patients to determine their choices

and act to improve their situation instead of only reacting.

I help my patients realize that even when they feel they have limited choices or little hope there is always a direction that allows a patient to be in control of their pain and therefore their outcome. I teach my patients that they get to choose how their pain and conditions define them. Patients that currently feel helpless are allowing their circumstances and conditions to control them. For example, a helpless patient may respond with "there's nothing I can do about my pain". I teach my patients to focus their time and energy on things they have control over. For example, my patients get to decide if they will wake up and do something productive today. They get to decide if they will interact positively with their family despite how their pain is making them feel. I help to teach my patients ways to empower their situation. That feeling of empowerment propels patients to gain more and more control of their pain. Focusing on items we do control instead of the items we can't control help to reduce stress levels which decrease anxiety and help my patients to better cope with their pain.

I teach patients to eliminate certain phrases including: "I can't", "I must", "If only", 'there's nothing I can do".

I help patients break the handcuffs of negativity that surround and influence their painful condition.

I help patients look at alternatives so that they can instead take a different approach and be in control, only then can you find an effective treatment plan for your pain.

# Get Moving!

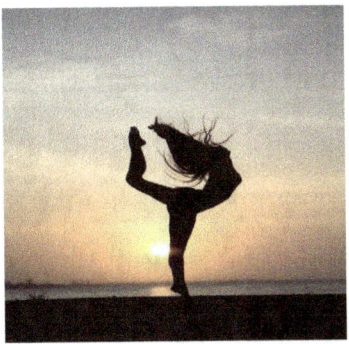

To effectively treat your pain, all patients need some level of an exercise routine. Obviously, many pain conditions can significantly limit the types of exercise a patient can perform but every patient can do some level activity above their sedentary status.

The gold standard exercise for chronic back pain patients is aquatic therapy. In fact most patients seem to respond to aquatic therapy as it is a way to improve range of motion, flexibility, and attain some level of cardiovascular workout in a controlled environment that is less stressful to the joints than land based activities.

Low impact yoga or some form of a daily stretching routine is another excellent form of daily exercise that almost all patients should add to their daily routine. Fibromyalgia patients seem to be a particular set of patients that I have personally witnessed make great strides.

For wheelchair bound patients, there are now excellent chair based exercise classes. In my 23 years of practice I've literally never found a patient that couldn't benefit from some type of exercise routine.

A daily exercise routine, improves strength and flexibility which can help patients avoid falls. Falls are very common with pain patients and can lead to further pain and disability. Daily exercise will improve a patient's mood and help them establish a positive routine to their day.

Check with your health care provider before starting an exercise routine. Afterwards, find some movement that you can stick with and perform most days of the week and get moving!

# Social Support

An often overlooked part of any patient's treatment plan is a friend to offer support. A friend, or some form of a supportive social network, is key to any recovery. This can range from a family member, an understanding neighbor, friend or online support group.

It's seems that for some of my pain patients I act as much a counselor rather than a traditional medical provider. Sometimes patients just simply need someone to vent their frustrations and aggravations to, someone who will take the time to listen and empathize with their situation. For some of my patients, a trip to the office is the highlight of their social calendar for the month.

I encourage all patients to find someone who they can spend quality time with in a supportive and caring manner. This social bond has an effective psychological impact on a patient's recovery. Having social support helps to motivate patients to be more active and involved. For some patients, their social network is severely limited due to their disability or lack of proximity to family and friends. Even patients with severe isolation issues can find some form of social network. I encourage home bound patients to join an online therapy or support group that is tailored to patients with their similar condition. This can be an effective tool to use as a sounding board for advice or support. Of course, always discuss any information gathered on these message boards with your local provider before implementing.

Find a friend who will listen and get involved!

# Laughter

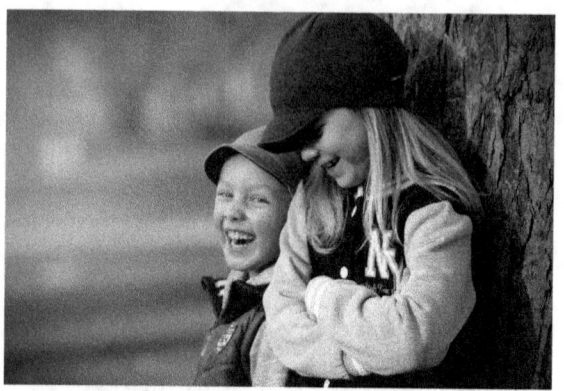

A very successful and overlooked tool in the treatment of chronic pain is laughter. Laughter holds many known benefits for the body from both a psychological and physiological perspective.

Laughter is known to lower blood pressure and reduce stress hormone levels. Laughter, the actual act of laughing, can also improve cardiac health. Laughter is known to improve immune function which is a vital factor in your recovery. Laughing also triggers the release of endorphins which are your body's natural pain killers. Laughing also improves a patient's general well being. Laughter improves circulation and smooth muscle relaxation, of vital importance to patient's suffering from chronic muscular pain conditions and ailments.

Beyond these physical responses to laughter, I have found that patients who regularly incorporate laughter have an improved outlook to their pain. Patient's who have the insight to laugh at their circumstances have improved quality of life and improved overall function. The old theory of the glass half full really does seem to apply to pain patients and helps to set realistic expectations.

So find a few moments every day to add some laughter back into your life.

# Crank up the Tunes!

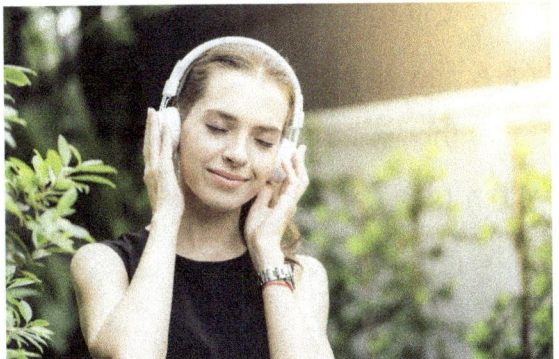

Music has the ability to be an amazing adjunctive therapy to help treat chronic pain. Neuroscientists have discovered that listening to music heightens positive emotion through stimulating dopamine levels. Dopamine has powerful effects on the reward center in the brain that affect emotion and pain control. Dopamine release from music has also been tied to improving motivation which helps gives pain patients the energy to be more active. Numerous studies have shown that athletes who train with music have improved endurance.

Music helps manage and control pain in a multitude of factors. Music has the ability to reduce stress and anxiety. Research shows music can prevent anxiety-induced increases in heart rate and high blood pressure. Listening to music can help reduce cortisol levels, a stress hormone. The power of music seems to act on both a physiological as well as psychological level to help patients better manage their pain. Music therapy is now being used as a means of conditioning patients to relax and release pain and stress.

So crank up your favorite tunes to decrease pain, improve mood, improve motivation and get yourself on the road to recovery.

# Work on your Sleep

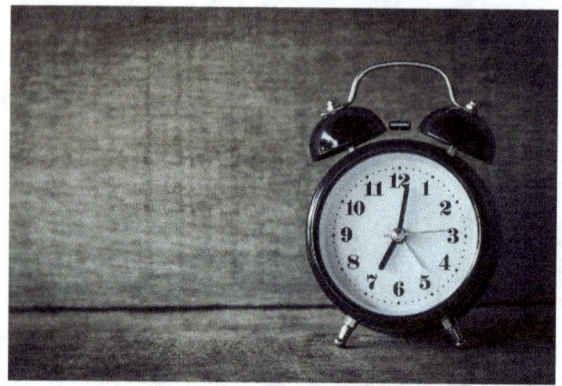

One common thread for the majority of pain patients is poor sleep. Yes, pain can keep patients from a good night sleep, but more and more studies are revealing that many pain conditions, specifically chronic pain conditions like Fibromyalgia are worsened by poor sleep patterns. Altered sleep patterns or poor sleep will impact the neurological, psychological, and physical function of the body. It has the same affect as a battery that never fully recharges.

I order sleep studies on all of my chronic pain patients. Many patients falsely believe that sleep studies are only valuable if a patient snores or has sleep apnea but this is false. Many patients have an underlying condition that has not been addressed. Sleep apnea can range from a true obstruction but can also pertain to patients that hold their breath while they sleep, so although they don't have a classic snore they still have poor perfusion of oxygen to the organs and this can directly impact the body's own healing mechanisms. Sleep studies can also identify what stages of sleep a patient is in the majority of the night. Most chronic pain patients and classically Fibromyalgia patients spend the majority of their night in lighter stages of sleep and never enter the deeper restorative phases. Impaired sleep can also exacerbate other chronic health conditions including Hypertension and Type 2 Diabetes.

A first step toward helping to treat your chronic pain is to rule out or treat any underlying sleep disturbances.

In later chapters I will discuss some effective medication and interventions to improve sleep.

# Rest

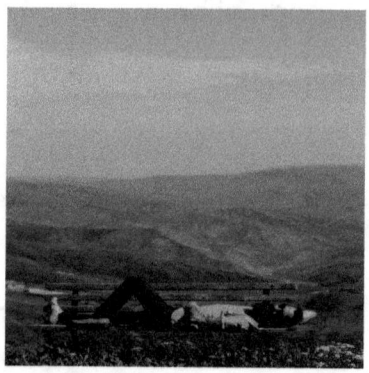

To help effectively treat your pain you must become more active and vigilant in your own recovery and yes this also applies to taking advantage of your rest. Rest come in many forms from improving your sleep, which we have already discussed, naps, meditation, stretching, and an approach to activity known as a active rest.

So much of our life seems to be some automated loop, whether that is our routine of running off to work in the morning or running our kids to school and various activities. People adapt to their hectic loop of a life by running from one activity to the next, pumping caffeine into their bodies at the local java hut to keep moving.

There is an argument that hitting the pause button and trying to find a better balance to our hectic lives and finding opportunities to rest is an excellent way to heal our body and our soul. A conscious approach to adding active rest based activities is a natural approach to living within your bodies circadian rhythm. Most research show that humans are designed to take an afternoon nap. Although a nap is not possible for most, finding 10 minutes to meditate or take a nature stroll seems to do wonders. For patients able to exercise, I recommend alternating between a heavy exercise day with a lighter exercise day to not over stress our body. For patients with more disabilities to activity, I recommend trying to stagger doctor appointments or busy days so as to not overwhelm yourself psychologically or physically.

I am not promoting a couch potato lifestyle rather I'm simply recognizing that making a conscious

decision to rest on the couch and
read a book or relax the mind
periodically is a healthy choice.

## Meditation

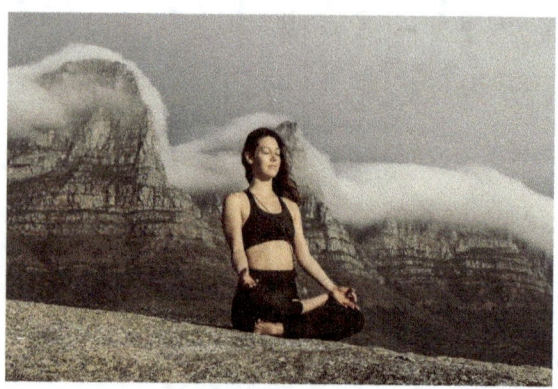

Meditation is an effective tool to help avoid additional prescription medications and help cure pain. Meditation can rewire the brain's pain circuitry. Neuronal pathways within the brain get programmed every time you expect pain to occur. In time, less and less stimulus is needed to trigger the pain reflex.

Eventually, the simple thought of pain becomes the true source, not necessarily the ailment itself.

Meditation can unhook your emotional reaction to pain. My patients can get stuck in a brutal feedback loop, without even realizing it. Their anticipation of pain creates stress, stress leads to physical tension within the body — especially near the painful area which ultimately leads to more pain.

Meditation teaches you how to emotionally detach from your negative thoughts and physical sensations, where you no longer expect pain, nor resist it when it does occur.

Meditation can also help us treat our natural flight or fight response to pain which can be abnormally triggered in chronic pain patients. The flight or fight increases cortisol stress levels. Elevated stress levels increase blood pressure, increase inflammatory markers and increase pain. Meditation helps to reduce these harmful stress hormone levels.

Meditation can also boost natural endorphin levels which act as a natural pain reliever, decrease cortisol levels and allow patients to be in control of their pain.

# Mindfulness

For motivated patients I encourage them to study and incorporate mindfulness into their daily routine. Mindfulness is the psychological process off bringing one's attention to experiences in the moment. It is best accomplished with training and the practice of meditation. Mindfulness interventions are effective in reducing rumination and worry. Rumination on one's pain or illness exacerbates depression and underlying anxiety conditions. A classic example is with my Fibromyalgia patients, they commonly ruminate on the condition and identify themselves as 'Fibro' instead of focusing on a more positive aspect of their life.

Classic mindfulness treatments I recommend to patients include a very basic mindfulness meditation where a patient sits and quietly focuses on their natural breathing. The patients are taught to allow thoughts to come and go without any judgement, simply allow the thoughts to dissolve away and then focus back on their breathing. A simple 3-5 minutes per day will start to show dramatic benefits in as little as 2 weeks as patients learn to wipe away anxiety and help to distract from the negative effects of pain on the mind.

A few apps that I have found helpful for patients to practice mindfulness include: Headspace, Aura and the app Stop Breath & Think.

As a patient incorporates a mindfulness approach to their daily routine, pain levels decrease, anxiety decreases, empowerment increases and patients inch closer to a more effective treatment for their pain.

# Spirituality

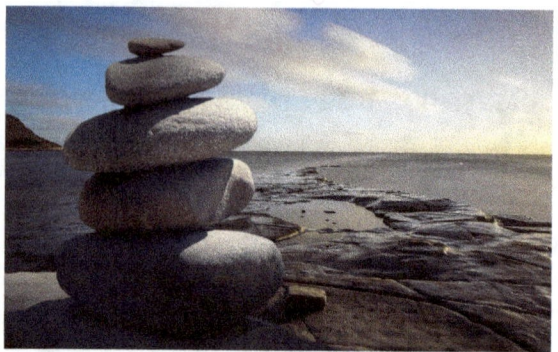

Chronic pain is a misunderstood
and complex condition to treat.
Research on the biology and
neurobiology of pain has shown a
relationship between spirituality and
pain. Using a number of cognitive
and behavioral strategies to cope
with pain, including religious/spiritual
factors, such as prayer or seeking
spiritual support to manage pain is

an essential component to finding an effective treatment for your pain.

Many patients confuse spirituality with religion. Although the two can overlap there is a difference between religion and spirituality. Religion is an organized faith system grounded in institutional practices while spirituality is grounded in personal beliefs and practices that can be expressed with or without a specific formal religious belief.

The role of spirituality in treating chronic pain is vital as it helps patients to create a meaning and purpose that is essential in fighting chronic pain. Spirituality can help patients cope with the physical as well as the psychological component to chronic pain. The psychological meaning that patients assign to their pain impacts how they process their pain long term.

Spirituality lies in the sense of connection and inner strength and peace that individuals derive from the relationship with themselves, others, nature and possibly a connection to a specific religion. The role of a more spiritual patient is vital to improving a patient's overall well-being and quality of life. This improved well being takes time and training to accomplish but works through visualization, meditation, positive thinking and possibly even prayer.

A sense of connection to one's environment, nature and a higher power helps to give patient's an improved outlook on their treatment and significantly improved outcomes in treating their pain. Patients that find the ability to improve their inner strength will have an improved outlook, a sense of purpose and will lead them to a more effective treatment and success managing their chronic pain.

# Food Intake

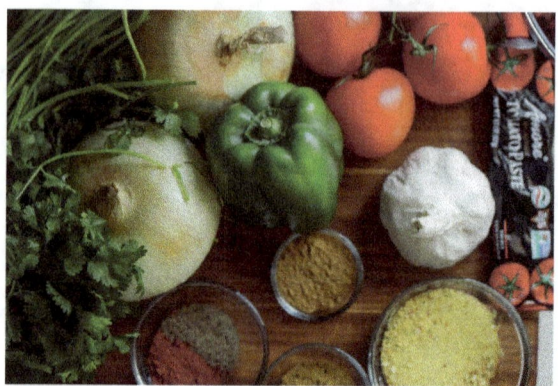

To make progress in finding an effective treatment for your pain, every patient needs to evaluate the food they put into their body. Your food is the fuel your body uses to heal and to repair itself. There are countless studies that show direct correlation to increased inflammatory levels and increased pain with different food groups.

Here is a list of foods I recommend to avoid or consider a 6 week elimination trial.

#1 Avoid all sodas! Interesting enough, diet soft drinks, due to the sweetener Aspartame, seem to have even worse detrimental side effects for pain patients. I have seen dramatic results from patients eliminating all soft drinks and replacing with water. Eliminating soft drinks improves energy, decreases inflammatory levels that trigger or exacerbate Migraine Headaches, joint pain and Fibromyalgia.

#2 Limit or eliminate "Night shade" plants. Most patients assume that increasing vegetables would be a good lifestyle choice, however increasing studies are revealing that pain patients do worse with exposure to nightshade plants. Nightshade plants include a list of vegetables including tomatoes, peppers, white potatoes, eggplant and more! These nightshade plants increase inflammatory levels in the body and increase pain.

#3 Limit Carbohydrates! Carbs, specifically yeast related products worsen pain and specifically for Fibromyalgia patients.

#4 Avoid Fast food, not even going to explain this further.

#5 Do your best to shop the outer ring of the grocery store. The outer ring of the grocery store will have more of the food that should be put into our body. The inner aisles contain all the processed foods. Obviously it's impossible to avoid all of the inner aisles, but if you start on the outer ring you will improve your nutritional value.

#6 Consider being evaluated for Gluten sensitivity or allergy.

This list will give you a good starting point to cleaning up your food intake and improving the food that fuels your body.

# Avoid Soda!

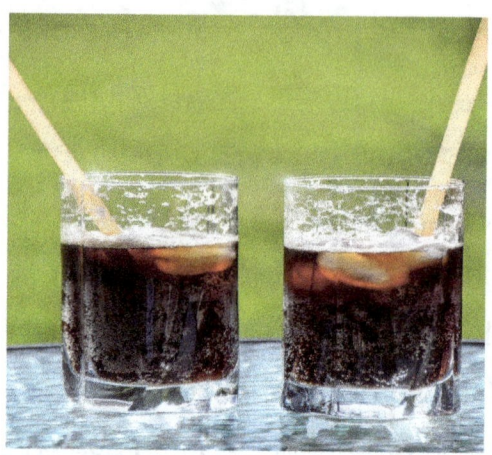

As discussed above, every patient with chronic pain will find tremendous improvement in eliminating soda.

The origins of soda drinks can be traced to a pharmacist that wanted to stimulate the brain by creating a mixture that contained cocaine. Despite the removal of the cocaine, though, many more drugs that activate the brain remain in these popular drinks like caffeine, sugar and flavor enhancers. More and more popular drinks are heavily loaded with caffeine, known to give people an energy boast and, when consumed regularly, these drinks also cause caffeine dependency.

The constant ups and downs of a caffeine roller coaster ride cause headaches, insomnia, mood instability and pain. Caffeine is a brain stimulant, a drug that can over-stimulate the brain and sometimes even cause death.

Sugar in soda is also a drug. Sugar not only stimulates the brain and causes dependency, it also harms the body in other ways. Complications from sugar include diabetes, a disease hallmarked by the harmful effects of frequent blood sugar spikes and consistently high blood sugar levels. Anyone who is experiencing pain should be extra cautious about avoiding anything that contains sugar because sugar promotes inflammation and inflammation leads to pain. In addition to sugar, sodas contain another, lesser known chemical that can lead to more pain, Aspartame. For years, researchers have reported about the potential harmful effects of Aspartame, a flavor enhancer. The effects are primarily seen in the nervous system such as: headaches, depression, anxiety and blurred vision. This chemical is meant to stimulate the taste buds but it appears to do more than that in some people. Aspartame could even contribute to a painful experience by sensitizing the nervous system.

Over the past 23 years, I have seen dramatic pain relief in patients who eliminate soda, specifically in patients who suffer from neuropathic pain and Fibromyalgia.

# Easy on the Carbs

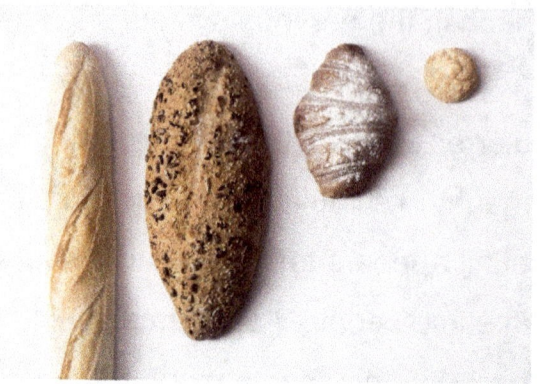

Carbohydrates make up the majority of the calories in many Americans' diets. Carbohydrates are a type of macro-nutrient which provide the body with energy. Grains such as bread, cereals, pasta and rices are all types of carbohydrates. Carbohydrates also come from fruits, vegetables and the natural sugars found in dairy products.

Some quick education on Carbs can help patients to have a better understanding of foods to be wary of in fighting chronic pain. Refined carbohydrates, such as white bread, white rice, cookies and candies, sodas, contain very little benefits to our general health. Refined carbs are low in fiber, vitamins and minerals. Complex carbohydrates such as whole wheat bread, brown rice, broccoli and asparagus, are rich in dietary fiber, help to stabilize blood sugar levels and are better choices for pain patients. Complex carbohydrates also contain high levels of vitamins and minerals.

Interesting enough most chronic pain patients, specifically Fibromyalgia patients, tend to have more frequent cravings for carbohydrates than healthy individuals. When patients give into the simple carbs they can enter a hypoglycemic state, or a sudden drop in blood sugar, perpetuating the fatigue and pain of Fibromyalgia and other chronic pain conditions.

Cutting out all carbohydrates from the diet is not recommended, since they do serve an important function in the metabolic process. Instead, I recommend cutting out all refined carbohydrates and choosing complex carbohydrates to make up 30% of your daily calorie intake.

These changes can significantly decrease inflammatory levels, improve energy and decrease pain.

## Avoid Fast Food

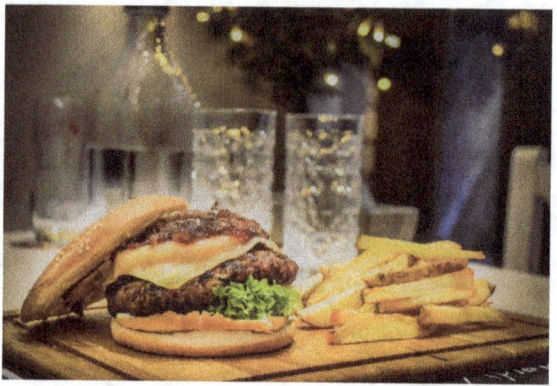

This is likely the most obvious of our recommendations for treating a patient's pain but also one of the most unlikely to be followed. Maybe it's our hectic lifestyle or just the fact that fast food is so cheap and convenient. Either way, patients inherently know that fast food is horrible for their general health and for pain but they just can't avoid it.

Fast food is not only quick to be prepared, but also contain some special group of fats that are known to be extremely harmful for the whole body, including for your joints. These fats, either saturated or trans can make the joints weaker and increase inflammatory markers. Alongside with trans and saturated fats, fast food contain high levels of sugar which also increases inflammatory markers and increases pain. Fast food also contains high levels of sodium, it is the main component of all non-organic pieces in a burger and usually it is the common ingredient that brings the whole taste to your meal.

Fast food with it's high levels of sodium, sugars, trans fats and carbohydrates combines to form what we like to call the pain bomb cocktail. This cocktail is further enhanced in Fibromyalgia patients as almost half Fibro patients suffer from Irritable Bowel Syndrome and leaky gut. Fast food also directly increases the likelihood of obesity and a sedentary lifestyle which in the long run will put more stress on joints and increase pain. Fast food will also increase the likeliness of heart disease and Type 2 Diabetes. Diabetic patients are at increased risk of peripheral neuropathies and chronic pain conditions.

Research an anti-inflammatory diet lifestyle and you will feel significantly better within a few weeks.

# Avoid Nicotine

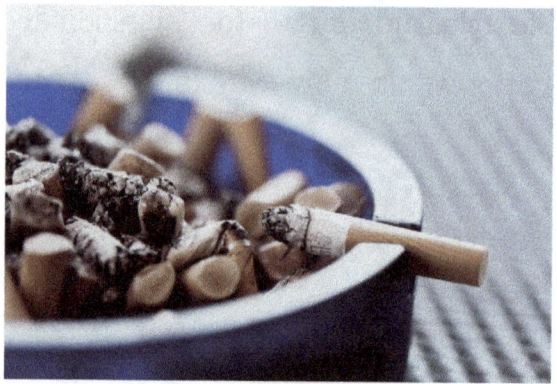

Over the past several years,
increasing numbers of medical
studies have shown the detrimental
and negative effects of cigarette use
and nicotine dependence on
multiple aspects of health regarding
the treatment of pain. Studies have
shown that cigarette smoking and all
other forms of nicotine consumption
worsens the results of virtually all

chronic pain treatments including cortisone injections and surgery. Also, everyone is well aware of the multitude of other health risks and expenses associated with nicotine consumption.

More recently, studies have shown an association between nicotine and the promotion of inflammation levels which directly worsen pain conditions and slow healing. Nicotine is a vasoconstrictor, shrinking blood vessels, which impacts oxygen perfusion to tissues and slows the body's own healing mechanisms and directly worsens pain and can led to further injury. Current research also reveals that nicotine acts as an accelerant to nerve related pain, similar to throwing gasoline on a fire.

Obviously, not all patients in pain use nicotine products, but roughly 60% do! If you want to find an effective treatment for your pain, you must first put down the nicotine so that you're not impeding your own recovery!

# Anxiety and Depression

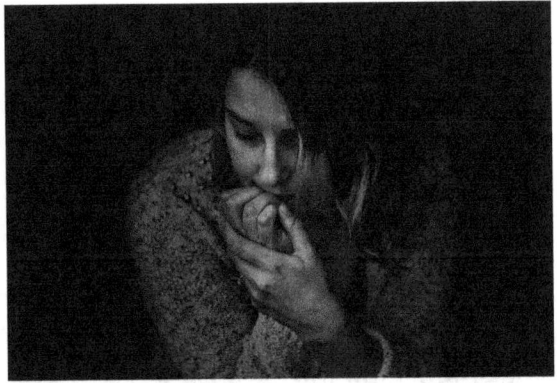

Chronic pain and depression are so closely linked that a viscous cycle can easily set in if one does not honestly address and treat any underlying depression. Studies show that patients with chronic pain have lower levels of the hormones serotonin and norepinephrine compared to patients not in pain. Lower levels of these hormones are known to lead to depression and anxiety. Combine these physiological lower levels of hormones with the frustration patient's feel regarding their lower quality of life and limitations from their pain and you have a set up for patients to fall into a feeling of hopelessness.

An important step towards finding an effective treatment for your pain is to work to attack depression directly. Depression is a medical condition that should be treated with a multi-modality approach. I work with our patients on setting up successful coping skills and techniques to improve their outlook on pain and depression. For a good amount of patients, working with a clinical psychologist or psychiatrist will also be a valuable member of a patient's pain fighting team. There are prescription medications that not only treat depression related issues but also have FDA indications for pain. Cymbalta is one example as it has FDA indications for Fibromyalgia, Diabetic peripheral neuropathy, chronic low back pain as well as anxiety and depression.

For patients that want to avoid traditional pharmacological medications, supplements like Magnesium have been used to treat stress and are an excellent smooth muscle relaxant. If you want to avoid pills all together, meditation and exercise are two successful strategies that every patient would benefit from. Both meditation and exercise boost endorphin levels, decrease stress hormone levels and give patients an improved outlook on life.

Finally, anyone with depression issues need to find someone to talk with, whether that be a support group, licensed professional, or a close friend. Releasing stress through the power of conversation is vital in helping patients gain both insight and learn tools to better cope with pain and depression.

# Traditional Pain Management

Pain management is a crucial aspect of healthcare that aims to relieve pain and improve quality of life for individuals suffering from chronic or acute pain. There has been significant advancement in pain management techniques over the years, and several approaches are currently used to manage pain, including pharmacological and non-pharmacological therapies. In the upcoming chapters I will provide an overview of the current pain management techniques.

Pharmacological therapies are the most commonly used pain

management techniques. Over-the-counter pain relievers, such as acetaminophen and ibuprofen, are commonly used for mild to moderate pain. For more severe pain, prescription medications, such as nonsteroidal anti-inflammatory drugs (NSAIDs), opioids, and anticonvulsants, may be used. These medications work by reducing the perception of pain, but they may also have side effects, such as drowsiness, stomach discomfort, and addiction.

Non-pharmacological therapies are becoming increasingly popular as they target the underlying cause of pain, rather than just reducing the perception of pain. Physical therapy, massage, acupuncture, and cognitive-behavioral therapy are some of the most commonly used non-pharmacological therapies. These therapies help to relieve pain by addressing muscle tension, emotional stress, and other factors that contribute to pain.

Interventional pain management techniques are another approach that involves the use of special devices or medications to target specific nerve pathways and relieve pain. Nerve blocks, epidural injections, and spinal cord stimulation are some of the most commonly used interventional techniques. These procedures can provide effective pain relief for individuals suffering from conditions such as chronic back pain, nerve pain, and other types of chronic pain.

Multidisciplinary pain management programs are becoming increasingly popular as they take a holistic approach to pain management. These programs involve a team of healthcare providers, including pain specialists, physical therapists, psychologists, and other professionals, who work together to provide individualized care for patients. Multidisciplinary programs can provide a range of treatments, including physical therapy, pain medications, and other therapies, to help individuals manage their pain.

Complementary and alternative therapies, such as herbal remedies, acupuncture, and massage, are also becoming increasingly popular for pain management. These therapies can provide natural and non-invasive ways to relieve pain, and they may be used in conjunction with other pain management techniques.

In conclusion, there are several effective pain management techniques currently used to relieve pain and improve quality of life for individuals suffering from chronic or acute pain. A combination of pharmacological and non-pharmacological therapies, along with interventional techniques and multidisciplinary programs, can provide effective pain relief and improve overall quality of life. It is important to work with a healthcare provider to determine the best approach for pain management and to ensure safe and effective pain relief. Below I will begin to dive into the various medical conditions and current treatment modalities.

# Fibromyalgia 101

Let's put to the side the past stigmas associated with Fibromyalgia. For many years a majority of physicians did not believe in Fibromyalgia and there are still a few physicians who refuse to recognize or treat Fibro patients. While rounding on patients in the hospital, I have overhead a colleague label Fibromyalgia as the "depressed, overweight, middle age, housewife syndrome".

Luckily, the medical community is finally coming around to recognizing this chronic pain condition. Current Fibromyalgia research and treatment philosophy resolves around the theory of Fibromyalgia being a mixed component of a central nervous system dysfunction with a chronic myofascial component.

Fibromyalgia is a diagnosis of exclusion.  It is important to make sure to have labs to rule our other connective tissues diseases first, like Rheumatoid Arthritis, before accepting the Fibro diagnosis.

Below is a list of recommendations I make to all of our Fibromyalgia patients on their first visit:

1.Every Fibro patient needs a sleep study to treat any underlying sleep disorders that will directly

complicate pain.

2.Treat any underlying depression,

this can not be understated!

Whether with counseling, psychiatric

treatment, meditation and if needed

medication

3.Check underlying vitamin

deficiencies that can complicate

pain, including Vitamin D, Vitamin

B12, Vitamin B1, Vitamin B2 and

Vitamin B6.

4.Start a daily home

exercise/stretching program, Fibro

will worsens with inactivity. I have

heard every argument from patients

that it hurts to much to exercise but

it is critical to do some daily

stretching/exercise routine. I
recommend low impact yoga,
pilates, tai chi, aquatic therapy.
5.Eliminate all soda's immediately,
totally toxic and can increase
inflammatory levels in the body
complicating pain.
6.Restrict the 'nightshade plants'
from the diet to limit their
inflammatory related issues.
7.Limit yeast foods, so many of our
patients struggle with this one but it
will dramatically improve your
energy
8.Work with a local physician and
consider one of the FDA approved
medications for Fibromyalgia:
Cymbalta and Lyrica.

9. Consider low dose naltrexone trial. LDN is a game changer! Naltrexone works at the glial cells in the nervous system to help decrease nerve sensitivity.

10.Consider a workup for gluten allergy.

# Migraines

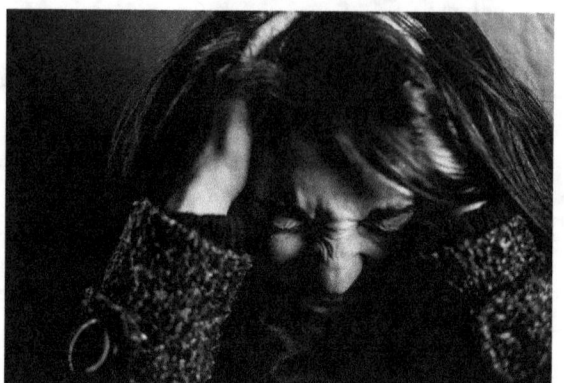

Migraine headaches are a common and debilitating condition that affects millions of people worldwide. Migraines are characterized by severe headaches, accompanied by a range of symptoms, including nausea, sensitivity to light and sound, and visual disturbances. The exact cause of migraines is not fully understood, but it is believed to be related to a combination of genetic and environmental factors.

There are several treatment options available for migraine headaches, including pharmacological and non-pharmacological therapies. In the next few chapters, I will provide an overview of the current treatment options for migraine headaches.

Pharmacological treatments for migraines are the most commonly used and include over-the-counter pain relievers, such as acetaminophen, and prescription medications, such as triptans and nonsteroidal anti-inflammatory drugs (NSAIDs). Triptans are a type of medication specifically designed to treat migraines, and they work by narrowing the blood vessels in the brain and reducing inflammation. NSAIDs, such as ibuprofen, can also be used to relieve migraine pain.

Preventative medications are also used to reduce the frequency and severity of migraines. These medications include beta-blockers, calcium channel blockers, and anticonvulsants, CGRP Inhibitors among others. Preventative medications can help to reduce the number of migraines a person experiences, making it easier to manage the condition.

Non-pharmacological treatments for migraines include lifestyle changes, such as regular exercise, stress management techniques, and dietary changes. Keeping a migraine diary can also be helpful in identifying triggers, such as certain foods or environmental factors, that may contribute to migraines.

Cognitive-behavioral therapy (CBT) and biofeedback are two forms of therapy that have been shown to be effective in managing migraines. CBT helps individuals to identify and manage negative thought patterns and behaviors that may contribute to migraines, while biofeedback helps individuals to understand and control the physical responses associated with migraines.

Interventional techniques, such as nerve blocks, SPG and Botox injections, may also be used to manage migraines. Nerve blocks are used to block pain signals to the brain, while Botox injections can help to relax the muscles that are associated with migraines.

Finally, complementary and alternative therapies, such as

acupuncture, massage, and herbal remedies, may also be used to manage migraines. These therapies can provide natural and non-invasive ways to relieve migraine pain and may be used in conjunction with other treatments.

In conclusion, there are several effective treatment options available for migraine headaches. A combination of pharmacological and non-pharmacological therapies, along with interventional techniques and complementary and alternative therapies, can provide effective relief for individuals suffering from migraines. It is important to work with a healthcare provider to determine the best approach for managing migraines and to ensure safe and effective pain relief.

# CGRP

CGRP inhibitors are a novel new treatment for Headaches

Calcitonin gene-related peptide (CGRP) is a neuropeptide that is involved in the regulation of pain, particularly in the management of headache disorders. Over the past few years, there has been a growing interest in the use of CGRP inhibitors as a treatment option for headaches, including migraines. This essay will provide a comprehensive overview of CGRP, its role in headaches, and the current status of CGRP-based treatments for headaches.

CGRP is a peptide hormone that is produced and released by sensory neurons in response to various triggers. It acts as a vasodilator, causing the blood vessels in the head to expand, leading to increased blood flow and inflammation. CGRP is also involved in the transmission of pain signals from the periphery to the central nervous system. It has been found to play a key role in the pathophysiology of migraines and other types of headaches.

There are two main types of CGRP inhibitors: monoclonal antibodies (mAbs) and small molecule drugs.

mAbs work by binding to CGRP in the bloodstream, preventing it from reaching the blood vessels and reducing inflammation. Small molecule drugs, on the other hand, block the CGRP receptors, preventing CGRP from binding and activating the receptors.

CGRP inhibitors have shown promise in the treatment of migraines and other types of headaches. Clinical trials have shown that CGRP inhibitors are effective in reducing the frequency and severity of migraines, as well as reducing the use of rescue medications. The benefits of CGRP inhibitors have also been demonstrated in patients with cluster headaches, a rare but debilitating form of headache.

One of the most promising CGRP inhibitors is erenumab (Aimovig), which is a monoclonal antibody that has been approved by the US Food and Drug Administration (FDA) for the treatment of migraines. Erenumab is administered as a subcutaneous injection and has been shown to reduce the frequency and severity of migraines by 50% or more in some patients. Another CGRP inhibitor, fremanezumab (Ajovy), has also been approved by the FDA for the treatment of migraines. It is administered as a subcutaneous injection and has been shown to reduce the frequency of migraines by 50% or more in some patients.

Small molecule CGRP inhibitors are also being developed and tested for the treatment of headaches. One of the most promising of these drugs is ubrogepant (Ubrelvy), which has been approved by the FDA for the treatment of acute migraines. Ubrogepant is taken orally and has been shown to provide rapid and effective relief from migraine symptoms.

In addition to the benefits in the management of headaches, CGRP inhibitors have also been shown to have positive effects on other conditions, such as cardiovascular disease and stroke. CGRP has been found to play a role in the development of these conditions, and the inhibition of CGRP may help to prevent or manage them.

Despite the promising results of CGRP inhibitors in the treatment of headaches, there are still some challenges that need to be addressed. One of the main challenges is the cost of CGRP inhibitors, which can be quite high.

The high cost may limit access to these treatments for many patients, especially those who do not have insurance coverage. Additionally, the long-term safety and efficacy of CGRP inhibitors are not yet fully understood, and further research is needed to fully understand their effects over the long-term.

# Botox for Migraine

Botulinum toxin type A, commonly known as Botox, is a popular and effective treatment option for individuals suffering from headaches. Botox works by temporarily blocking the release of chemicals that transmit pain signals in the brain. This reduces the frequency and severity of headaches, providing relief for individuals who suffer from chronic migraines, tension headaches, and other types of headaches. In this essay, we will provide an overview of the current uses of Botox for headache treatment and its potential benefits and risks.

Botox has been used as a treatment for headaches for over two decades, and its effectiveness has been widely documented in numerous clinical studies. The American Migraine Foundation and the American Academy of Neurology have both endorsed the use of Botox for the treatment of chronic migraines. Botox is typically administered through a series of injections into specific muscle groups, and the treatment usually takes less than 30 minutes. The effects of Botox can last for up to three months, and the treatment can be repeated as needed.

One of the primary benefits of Botox for headache treatment is its ability to reduce the frequency and severity of headaches. In clinical studies, individuals who received Botox injections for their headaches experienced a significant reduction in the number of headaches per month compared to those who received a placebo. Additionally, Botox has been shown to improve quality of life and reduce the use of other headache medications, such as pain relievers and triptans.

Another benefit of Botox for headache treatment is its low risk profile. Botox has been used for cosmetic purposes for over 20 years and has a well-established safety record. The most common side effects of Botox for headache treatment are mild, such as temporary muscle weakness or soreness at the injection site, and they typically resolve on their own within a few days. Serious side effects are rare, but as with any medical procedure, it is important to discuss potential risks with a healthcare provider before undergoing treatment.

It is important to note that Botox is not a cure for headaches, but rather a tool for managing symptoms.

Individuals who receive Botox for their headaches may still experience occasional headaches, but the frequency and severity of these headaches are usually significantly reduced. Additionally, Botox does not work for everyone, and some individuals may not experience the full benefits of treatment.

In conclusion, Botox is a safe and effective treatment option for individuals suffering from headaches. Its ability to reduce the frequency and severity of headaches, improve quality of life, and low risk profile make it an attractive option for those seeking relief from chronic migraines, tension headaches, and other types of headaches. As with any medical procedure, it is important to discuss the potential benefits and risks with a healthcare provider and to determine the best approach for managing headaches. With ongoing research and advancements in headache treatment, Botox will likely continue to play a significant role in the management of headaches for years to come.

# SPG

The sphenopalatine ganglion (SPG) is a group of nerve cells located in the back of the nasal cavity that is believed to play a significant role in the development of certain types of headaches. The SPG has been targeted for treatment in recent years due to its potential for providing relief for headaches, including migraines and cluster headaches. In this essay, we will provide an overview of the current treatments for headaches using SPG stimulation.

One of the most common methods of SPG stimulation is a procedure called the Sphenopalatine Ganglion (SPG) Block. This is a minimally invasive procedure that involves the injection of a local anesthetic into the nasal cavity to block the SPG and provide relief from headaches. This procedure is typically performed in an outpatient setting and can provide quick relief for headache pain.

Another method of SPG stimulation is through the use of a device called the transcutaneous SPG (t-SPG) stimulator. This device is worn over the face and uses electrical stimulation to activate the SPG and provide relief from headaches. The t-SPG stimulator has been shown to be effective in reducing the frequency and severity of headaches and is a non-invasive alternative to the SPG block.

In addition to these techniques, a number of medications have been developed to target the SPG and provide relief from headaches. These medications, known as SPG-targeted drugs, work by blocking the SPG and reducing the frequency and severity of headaches. These drugs are typically administered through a nasal spray or other similar method and are used to provide long-term relief from headaches.

Another method of SPG stimulation involves the use of nerve stimulation techniques. This involves the use of a device that delivers electrical stimulation to the SPG, providing relief from headaches. This technique has been shown to be effective in reducing the frequency and severity of headaches and is a non-invasive alternative to other SPG stimulation techniques.

Finally, lifestyle changes, such as regular exercise, stress management techniques, and dietary changes, may also be effective in reducing the frequency and severity of headaches and may be used in conjunction with SPG stimulation techniques.

In conclusion, SPG stimulation is a promising new approach for the treatment of headaches, including migraines and cluster headaches. There are a number of techniques available, including the SPG block, t-SPG stimulation, SPG-targeted drugs, nerve stimulation techniques, and lifestyle changes, that can be used to provide relief from headaches. It is important to work with a healthcare provider to determine the best approach for managing headaches and to ensure safe and effective pain relief. With the ongoing development of new techniques and treatments, the future of SPG stimulation for headache treatment looks bright, offering new hope for individuals suffering from headaches.

I have seen SPG as a very successful treatment not only for headaches but various atypical facial pains, cluster headaches and even trigeminal neuralgia

## Sleep treatments

Sleep and pain management are intricately connected, with poor sleep often leading to increased pain and chronic pain causing disruptions to sleep. Studies have shown that individuals with chronic pain are more likely to experience poor sleep quality, and individuals with poor sleep quality are more likely to experience chronic pain.

Pain can interfere with sleep by causing discomfort, making it difficult to find a comfortable position, and causing frequent waking. In turn, sleep deprivation can lead to increased pain sensitivity, and can make it difficult for the body to effectively manage and cope with pain.

To address this connection, effective pain management strategies must include addressing sleep quality. This can be done through sleep hygiene practices, such as establishing a regular sleep schedule, creating a relaxing bedtime routine, and minimizing exposure to electronic devices before bedtime.

In addition, behavioral therapies, such as cognitive behavioral therapy for insomnia (CBT-I), can be effective in addressing both sleep and pain. CBT-I helps individuals change negative thought patterns and behaviors that contribute to sleep disturbances, and can help improve sleep quality, reduce pain, and improve overall quality of life.

Medications can also be used to treat sleep disturbances and pain. Sleep aids, such as benzodiazepines or non-benzodiazepine hypnotics, can help individuals fall asleep and stay asleep. Pain relievers, such as nonsteroidal anti-inflammatory drugs (NSAIDs) or opioids, can help reduce pain. However, it is important to use medications only as prescribed, and to discuss the potential risks and benefits with a healthcare provider.

It is important to treat any underlying conditions impacting sleep or quality of sleep. A significant majority of pain patients should undergo a formal sleep study to identify conditions.

An exciting new class of medication

includes the Orexin receptor medications.  They are a relatively new class of drugs that have shown promise in the treatment of sleep disorders. These medications work by targeting the orexin system in the brain, which is responsible for regulating wakefulness and sleep.

By blocking the actions of orexin, these medications can promote sleep and improve sleep quality in people with insomnia and other sleep disorders.

Clinical trials have shown the ability to significantly reduce the time it takes to fall asleep and increase total sleep time. It has also been found to have a favorable safety profile and low risk of dependency or abuse. Examples in this class of medication I use in practice include Dayvigo and Belsomra.

In conclusion, sleep and pain management are interrelated, and addressing one can often have a positive impact on the other.

Effective pain management strategies must include addressing sleep quality through sleep hygiene practices, behavioral therapies, and medications, as appropriate. By treating both pain and sleep, individuals can experience improved sleep quality and reduced pain, leading to improved overall quality of life.

# Mechanical Low Back Pain

A significant amount of chronic pain patients deal with chronic low back pain. This is a massive topic that I will give an overview to here and further breakdown in their own chapters. Mechanical back pain which is separate from discogenic back pain. The two main types of mechanical (axial) back pain are Sacroiliac Joint Dysfunction (SI Dysfunction) and Lumbar Spondylosis.

The Sacroiliac Joints are a pair of joints as the iliac crest attaches on either side of the sacrum, which is the bone just above your tailbone.

Patients with SI pain can have bilateral or unilateral pain. SI joint patients typically have trouble walking up inclines, getting up from a seated position and the pain is a complex combination of instability in the SI joint, inflammation and many times associated piriformis tendon involvement. There are physical therapists that spend their entire careers focused on treating SI joint pain and the therapy for SI dysfunction is completely different than physical therapy for common low back pain. When patients plateau with physical therapy we have found tremendous success in targeted interventional injections to the SI region. We will typically begin worth a combination of cortisone and anesthetic to work as both a diagnostic as well as therapeutic treatment. Patients who experience only limited benefits from this treatment are then likely candidates for prolotherapy to the region which is a specific series of injections designed to harness our body's own natural healing process. This is particularly helpful in patients who have an underlying instability in their SI joint.

For patient that continue to suffer from SI related pain, there are minimally invasive procedures to help stabilize the SI joint that can be done in an outpatient ambulatory surgery center. I have found both the PainTeq and CornerLoc procedure to be effective in tough to treat SI patients.

Lumbar Spondylosis is medical terminology for pain emanating from the facet joints in the vertebrae. The facet joints run on the back portion of the spine and we describe them as the 'knuckle' joints of the spine. They allow the spine to twist and move and are classic causes of back pain anywhere along the spine but a very common cause of low back pain. Classically, patients with facetogenic back pain describe pain with extension or rotation activities, standing to wash dishes and lifting activities. Many time patients will describe a catching sensation or will describe back pain that runs from the spine out along the belt line. As always I recommend a trial of physical therapy and various other modalities I have discussed in previous chapters. If patients fail all more conservative treatment I will consider facet joint injections. If the facet joints injections help but are only temporary I will then consider Radiofrequency Ablation injection to the affected facets. RF injections have a typical period of relief from 6-12 months.

The goal of these treatments are to improve function, decrease pain and hopefully avoid surgery. As always, diet, exercise, weight management, stress reduction are all integral in helping to improve any treatments.

# Radiofrequency

Radiofrequency facet ablation is a minimally invasive procedure used to treat chronic back pain that originates from the facet joints in the spine. Facet joints are small joints located between adjacent vertebrae that help stabilize the spine and facilitate movement. When these joints become inflamed or irritated, they can cause significant pain and discomfort. Radiofrequency facet ablation involves using a specialized needle to deliver a small electrical current to the affected joint, which heats and destroys the nerve fibers that transmit pain signals. The

Radiofrequency facet ablation is typically performed on an outpatient basis and takes about 30-60 minutes to complete. Patients are given local anesthesia and may be sedated to help them relax during the procedure. After the procedure, patients may experience some mild discomfort and soreness at the site of the injection, but this usually resolves within a few days. Most patients are able to resume their normal activities within a day or two, and many experience significant pain relief within a few weeks of the procedure. Most insurance covers this treatment every 6 months if necessary.

## Discogenic Pain

Discogenic pain is a type of chronic low back pain that originates from the intervertebral discs, the spongy cushions that sit between the vertebrae in the spine. Discogenic pain is thought to be caused by damage or degeneration of the discs, which can cause inflammation, nerve irritation, and muscle spasms. The pain is typically described as a deep, aching pain that is worse with prolonged sitting or standing, and may be accompanied by stiffness, numbness, or tingling in the legs.

Current treatment options for discogenic pain include both non-surgical and surgical approaches. Non-surgical treatments may include:

1. Physical therapy: Exercises and stretches can help improve flexibility and strength, and can also help alleviate pain.

2. Medications: Over-the-counter pain relievers, such as acetaminophen or nonsteroidal anti-inflammatory drugs (NSAIDs), may help relieve pain and reduce inflammation.

The Patient's Guide to Pain Management

3. Injections: Epidural steroid injections or nerve blocks may be used to provide temporary pain relief and potentially long term relief.

4. Chiropractic or massage therapy: These treatments may help alleviate pain and improve function.

# Sciatica

Sciatica is a type of low back pain that is caused by irritation or compression of the sciatic nerve, which runs from the lower back down to the legs. Non-surgical treatments for sciatica typically aim to alleviate pain, reduce inflammation, and improve function. Some of the most common non-surgical treatments for sciatica include:

1. Physical therapy: Exercises and stretches can help improve flexibility and strength, and can also help alleviate pain.

2. Medications: Over-the-

counter pain relievers, such as acetaminophen or nonsteroidal anti-inflammatory drugs (NSAIDs), may help relieve pain and reduce inflammation. In some cases, stronger prescription medications may be necessary. I have found success with Lyrica and Neurontin for neuropathic radicular pain relief.

3. Injections: Epidural steroid injections, or nerve blocks may be used to provide temporary and or long term pain relief. Insurance will classically cover up to 3-4

epidurals if needed.

4. Viadisc is an exciting new treatment for disc related disease.

# Viadisc

Viadisc is a non-surgical treatment option for patients with chronic low back pain caused by degenerative disc disease (DDD). DDD is a condition in which the intervertebral discs, which act as cushions between the vertebrae in the spine, degenerate over time, causing pain and other symptoms.

Viadisc involves the injection of a hydrogel into the affected disc, which can help restore the disc's height and cushioning properties. The hydrogel is composed of a biocompatible, water-based material that is designed to mimic the properties of natural intervertebral discs.

The procedure is typically performed on an outpatient basis under local anesthesia. A small needle is inserted into the affected disc under guidance of fluoroscopy or other imaging modalities, and the hydrogel is injected into the disc. The hydrogel then expands and forms a gel-like substance that provides cushioning and support to the disc.

Viadisc is intended for use in patients with mild to moderate DDD who have not responded to non-surgical treatments such as physical therapy, medications, or injections. The procedure is minimally invasive and has a relatively low risk of complications.

While the long-term effectiveness of Viadisc is still being evaluated through clinical trials, early results suggest that it may be a promising treatment option for some patients with chronic low back pain caused by DDD.

# Epidural Steroid Injections

Epidural steroid injections (ESIs) are a common procedure to place a dose of a steroid medication into the epidural space, which is the space surrounding the spinal cord and nerve roots.

ESIs are typically performed on an outpatient basis under local anesthesia or light sedation. A small needle is inserted into the epidural space under guidance of fluoroscopy or other imaging modalities, and the steroid medication is injected into the affected area. The medication then spreads throughout the epidural space and helps reduce inflammation and pain.

ESIs are commonly used to treat conditions such as herniated discs, spinal stenosis, and sciatica. The procedure can provide temporary relief from pain and inflammation, which may allow patients to participate in physical therapy or other treatments.

# Lumbar Stenosis

Spinal stenosis is a condition in which the spinal canal narrows, which can put pressure on the spinal cord and nerves, leading to pain, numbness, and weakness in the back, legs, or arms. The condition is most commonly caused by degenerative changes in the spine, such as arthritis or bulging discs.

Non-surgical treatment options for spinal stenosis typically aim to alleviate pain and improve function. Some of the most common non-surgical treatments for spinal stenosis include:

1. Physical therapy: Exercises and stretches can help improve flexibility and strength, and can also help alleviate pain.

2. Medications: Over-the-counter pain relievers, such as acetaminophen or nonsteroidal anti-inflammatory drugs (NSAIDs), may help relieve pain and reduce inflammation. In some cases, stronger prescription medications may be necessary.

3. Injections: Epidural steroid injections, facet joint injections, or nerve blocks

may be used to provide temporary pain relief.

4. Chiropractic or massage therapy: These treatments may help alleviate pain and improve function.

5. Assistive devices: Braces, canes, or walkers may help support the back and improve mobility.

# Vertiflex

Vertiflex is a minimally invasive, outpatient procedure that is used as an alternative to traditional spine surgery for lumbar stenosis. Lumbar stenosis is a condition in which the spinal canal in the lower back narrows, causing compression of the nerves and leading to pain, weakness, and other symptoms.

The Vertiflex procedure involves the insertion of a small, titanium alloy spacer between the affected vertebrae in the lower back. The spacer is designed to maintain the space between the vertebrae, relieving pressure on the nerves and reducing symptoms.

The procedure is typically performed under local anesthesia, and patients can typically return home the same day. Recovery time is generally shorter than with traditional spine surgery, and most patients are able to resume normal activities within a few weeks.

The Vertiflex procedure is most appropriate for patients with moderate to severe lumbar stenosis who have not responded to other non-surgical treatments. It is also suitable for patients who may not be able to tolerate traditional spine surgery due to underlying health conditions or other factors.

I have found that Vertiflex is an excellent option for patients with 1 or 2 level stenosis and are trying to avoid larger neurosurgical options that come with higher risk and a more extended recovery period.

# Spinal Cord Stimulation

Spinal cord stimulation (SCS) is a medical treatment that uses a device to deliver low-level electrical stimulation to the spinal cord, which can help alleviate chronic pain. The device consists of small electrodes that are implanted under the skin near the spinal cord and a battery-powered generator that delivers the electrical impulses.

SCS is typically used to treat chronic pain that has not responded to other treatments, such as medication, physical therapy, or surgery. The most common conditions that SCS is used to treat include back and leg pain, neck and arm pain, and neuropathic pain.

The effectiveness of SCS varies depending on the individual patient and the underlying cause of the pain. Studies have shown that SCS can provide significant pain relief for many patients, with some experiencing up to 70% reduction in pain levels. SCS may also improve physical function and quality of life for some patients.

Before being approved for a SCS implant, patients will undergo an SCS trial during which a temporary electrode will be placed for 5-7 days to help determine if a patient is a candidate for implant.

Our office currently uses multiple SCS companies including Boston Scientific and Nevro. Nevro is a very interesting company as their HFX technology is the first to gain FDA indication for Diabetic Peripheral Neuropathy and for non surgical low back pain. Those 2 indications have been game changers and opened up SCS to a larger range of patients.

# Peripheral Neuropathy

Painful peripheral neuropathy is a condition in which there is damage to the nerves that carry signals from the extremities, such as the feet and hands, to the spinal cord and brain. This damage can result in chronic pain, numbness, tingling, and weakness in the affected areas.

The most common causes of painful peripheral neuropathy include diabetes, chemotherapy, alcoholism, and autoimmune disorders. Treatment options for painful peripheral neuropathy aim to alleviate symptoms and improve function, and may include:

1. Medications: Medications such as gabapentin, pregabalin(Lyrica), and duloxetine (Cymbalta) may be used to relieve pain, numbness, and tingling associated with peripheral neuropathy. Personally I have found that a combination of both Lyrica and Cymbalta is necessary for my complex peripheral neuropathy patients. Topical medications, such as lidocaine patches or capsaicin cream, may also provide relief but are definitely a second line treatment.

2. Physical therapy: Exercises and stretches can help improve muscle strength and flexibility, and may also help alleviate pain.

3. Transcutaneous electrical nerve stimulation (TENS): TENS is a treatment that uses a small device to deliver electrical impulses to the affected area, which can help alleviate pain.

4. Acupuncture: This involves the insertion of thin needles into specific points on the body, which can help alleviate pain and improve function.

5. Nutritional supplements: Supplements such as vitamin B12 and alpha-lipoic acid may help improve nerve function and alleviate symptoms.

6. Cognitive behavioral therapy (CBT): CBT can help patients learn coping strategies for managing chronic pain associated with peripheral neuropathy.

7. Spinal Cord Stimulation, especially Nevro's HFX technology, is now an effective treatment option.

8. RealWave PT is a new option

for peripheral neuropathy that
is FDA indicated but
somewhat limited as there
are currently only a few
RealWave Centers.

# Knee Osteoarthritis

Knee osteoarthritis (OA) is a common condition in which the protective cartilage in the knee joint breaks down, causing pain, swelling, and stiffness. While knee replacement surgery is often necessary for advanced cases, there are several nonsurgical pain treatments that can help manage symptoms and improve function. These may include:

1. Physical therapy: A physical therapist can work with patients to develop an exercise program that can help strengthen the muscles around the knee joint and

improve flexibility and
mobility.

2. Weight management: Excess
   weight can put extra stress
   on the knee joint,
   exacerbating symptoms of
   knee OA. Weight loss through
   diet and exercise can help
   alleviate pain and improve
   function.

3. Medications: Over-the-
   counter pain relievers such
   as acetaminophen or
   nonsteroidal anti-
   inflammatory drugs (NSAIDs)
   can help alleviate pain and
   inflammation associated with
   knee OA. Prescription

medications, such as corticosteroids or hyaluronic acid injections, may also be used to manage symptoms.

4. Bracing: A knee brace can help provide support and stability to the knee joint, which can alleviate pain and improve function.

5. Topical treatments: Creams, gels, or patches containing capsaicin or menthol may help alleviate pain associated with knee OA.

6. Viscosupplementation has been a very effective treatment for knee OA and

deserves it's own chapter.

7. PRP, which will deserve it's own chapter to follow as well.

# Viscosupplementation

Viscosupplementation is a nonsurgical treatment option for knee osteoarthritis (OA) that involves injecting a gel-like substance called hyaluronic acid into the knee joint. Hyaluronic acid is a naturally occurring substance in the body that helps lubricate and cushion the joints.

In patients with knee OA, the natural levels of hyaluronic acid in the synovial fluid that surrounds the knee joint are reduced, which can lead to pain and stiffness. Viscosupplementation aims to restore the natural levels of hyaluronic acid in the joint, thereby reducing pain and improving joint function.

The procedure involves injecting the hyaluronic acid gel directly into the knee joint using a needle. The injection is typically performed in a healthcare provider's office and takes only a few minutes. Patients may experience some discomfort during the injection, but this is usually mild and temporary.

The effects of viscosupplementation typically last for six to 12 months and is covered by insurance to be performed every 6 months if necessary. When describing viscosupplementation to patients I like to describe it as "putting WD40 on a squeaky wheel" as we are trying to increase lubrication and to decrease friction/inflammation.

# PRP

Platelet-rich plasma (PRP) is a nonsurgical treatment option for knee osteoarthritis (OA) that involves injecting a concentrated solution of a patient's own blood platelets into the affected knee joint. Platelets contain growth factors that can stimulate tissue repair and regeneration.

To prepare PRP, a healthcare provider will draw a small amount of the patient's blood and process it to concentrate the platelets. The resulting PRP solution is then injected into the knee joint using a needle.

PRP injections are typically performed in a healthcare provider's office and take only a few minutes. Patients may experience some discomfort during the injection, but this is usually mild and temporary.

The effects of PRP injections can vary depending on the severity of knee OA and the individual patient. Some patients may experience a reduction in pain and inflammation, as well as improvements in joint function and mobility. The effects of PRP injections may last for several months if not longer. The biggest downside to PRP has been that traditional insurance still views PRP as an 'alternative treatment' and so

because of the alternative
designation it does fall in to the self
pay category of treatment options.

# RSD

RSD (Reflex Sympathetic Dystrophy), also known as CRPS (Complex Regional Pain Syndrome), is a chronic pain condition that usually affects a single limb. It typically occurs after an injury or trauma and is characterized by severe pain, swelling, and changes in skin color and temperature.

The exact cause of RSD is unknown, but it is believed to result from an abnormal response of the sympathetic nervous system to the injury or trauma. The sympathetic nervous system is responsible for controlling many involuntary body functions, such as heart rate, blood pressure, and sweating. In RSD, the sympathetic nervous system becomes overactive, causing pain, swelling, and other symptoms.

There is currently no cure for RSD, but there are several treatment options available to help manage the symptoms. These include:

1. Medications: I may prescribe a variety of medications to help manage the pain associated with RSD. These can include nonsteroidal anti-inflammatory drugs (NSAIDs), corticosteroids, opioids,

antidepressants and anti-

seizure meds like like Lyrica

or Neurontin.

2. Physical therapy: Physical

therapy can help improve

range of motion, reduce pain,

and prevent muscle atrophy.

This may involve exercises to

strengthen the affected limb,

as well as stretching and

massage.

3. Sympathetic nerve blocks: In

some cases, doctors may

recommend a sympathetic

nerve block. This involves

injecting an anesthetic

medication directly into the

affected nerves to block the

overactive sympathetic nervous system.

4. Spinal cord stimulation: This involves the implantation of a small device that sends electrical impulses to the spinal cord, which can help reduce pain and improve function.

5. Psychological treatment: cognitive-behavioral therapy, to help cope with the emotional impact of the condition.

6. IV Ketamine has also been an exciting addition to the practice that has shown

sustained benefit for RSD.

It is important to note that the effectiveness of these treatments can vary depending on the severity of the condition and the individual patient's response. A multidisciplinary approach to treatment that involves a team of healthcare professionals may be necessary to manage the complex symptoms associated with RSD.

# Tennis Elbow

Tennis elbow, also known as lateral epicondylitis, is a painful condition that affects the tendons in the elbow, causing pain and inflammation. It is typically caused by repetitive motions, such as those used in racquet sports or manual labor, which can strain the tendons in the forearm that attach to the lateral epicondyle, a bony bump on the outer side of the elbow.

The symptoms of tennis elbow include pain and tenderness on the outer side of the elbow, weakness in the forearm, and difficulty gripping or lifting objects.

The treatment options for tennis elbow typically include:

1. Rest and ice: Resting the affected arm and applying ice to the area can help reduce pain and inflammation.

2. Physical therapy: Physical therapy can help strengthen the muscles and tendons in the forearm, as well as improve range of motion and flexibility.

3. Nonsteroidal anti-inflammatory drugs (NSAIDs): Medications such as ibuprofen or naproxen can help reduce pain and

inflammation. Including topical diclofenac.

4. Bracing or splinting: Wearing a brace or splint can help support the affected arm and reduce strain on the tendons.

5. Corticosteroid injections: In some cases, a corticosteroid injection may be given directly into the affected area to help reduce inflammation and pain.

6. Extracorporeal shockwave therapy (ESWT): ESWT is a non-invasive procedure that uses shock waves to stimulate the healing process

and reduce pain.

7. PRP treatments have been very effective in more difficult cases.

8. Surgery: In rare cases where other treatments have not been effective, surgery may be necessary to repair or remove damaged tissue.

# Carpal Tunnel Syndrome

Carpal Tunnel Syndrome (CTS) is a condition that affects the wrist and hand, caused by pressure on the median nerve which runs through the wrist, in a space called the carpal tunnel. It can cause pain, tingling, and numbness in the hand and fingers, particularly the thumb, index, and middle fingers.

The condition is usually caused by repetitive motions of the hand and wrist or other activities that involve flexing or extending the wrist repeatedly, which can cause swelling in the wrist and put pressure on the median nerve.

The treatment options for Carpal Tunnel Syndrome include:

1. Rest and wrist immobilization: Reducing the use of the affected hand and wrist and wearing a splint or brace to immobilize the wrist can help reduce pressure on the median nerve.

2. Physical therapy: Stretching and strengthening exercises can help improve wrist and hand function and reduce symptoms.

3. Nonsteroidal anti-inflammatory drugs (NSAIDs): Medications such as

ibuprofen or naproxen can
help reduce pain and
inflammation.

4. Corticosteroid injections: In
some cases, a corticosteroid
injection may be given
directly into the affected area
to help reduce inflammation
and pain.

5. Surgery: In severe cases,
surgery may be
recommended to relieve
pressure on the median
nerve. The most common
type of surgery for Carpal
Tunnel Syndrome is called
carpal tunnel release, which
involves cutting the ligament

that is pressing on the
median nerve to relieve
pressure.

6. Lifestyle changes: Changing
certain habits such as
avoiding repetitive motions,
taking breaks to rest and
stretch, and modifying work
activities can help prevent
recurrence of Carpal Tunnel
Syndrome.

# Plantar Fasciitis

Plantar fasciitis is a condition that causes pain and inflammation in the plantar fascia, a thick band of tissue that runs across the bottom of the foot, connecting the heel bone to the toes. It is a common condition that can affect people of all ages, but it is particularly common in runners and other athletes, as well as those who spend a lot of time on their feet.

The nonsurgical treatment options for plantar fasciitis include:

1. Rest and ice: Resting the affected foot and applying ice to the area can help reduce

pain and inflammation.

2. Stretching exercises: Stretching exercises can help improve flexibility and reduce tension in the plantar fascia.

3. Nonsteroidal anti-inflammatory drugs (NSAIDs): Medications such as ibuprofen or naproxen can help reduce pain and inflammation.

4. Orthotics: Wearing shoes with good arch support or using orthotic inserts can help reduce stress on the plantar fascia.

5. Physical therapy: Physical

therapy can help improve flexibility, strength, and range of motion in the foot and ankle.

6. Night splints: Wearing a night splint that keeps the foot and ankle in a neutral position can help reduce morning pain and stiffness.

7. Extracorporeal shockwave therapy (ESWT): ESWT is a non-invasive procedure that uses shock waves to stimulate the healing process and reduce pain.

8. Platelet-rich plasma (PRP) therapy: PRP therapy

involves injecting a

concentration of the patient's

own blood platelets into the

affected area to promote

healing.

# Shoulder Pain

There are several common shoulder pain conditions, including:

1. Rotator cuff tendinitis: Inflammation of the tendons in the rotator cuff can cause pain and weakness in the shoulder.

2. Bursitis: Inflammation of the bursa, a fluid-filled sac that cushions the joint, can cause pain and tenderness in the shoulder.

3. Frozen shoulder: Also known as adhesive capsulitis, frozen shoulder is a condition in which the shoulder joint

becomes stiff and painful, making it difficult to move.

4. Shoulder impingement syndrome: This condition occurs when the tendons in the rotator cuff become trapped and compressed between the bones in the shoulder, causing pain and weakness.

The nonsurgical treatment options for these conditions include:

1. Rest and ice: Resting the affected shoulder and applying ice to the area can help reduce pain and inflammation.

2. Physical therapy: Physical therapy can help improve flexibility, strength, and range of motion in the shoulder.

3. Nonsteroidal anti-inflammatory drugs (NSAIDs): Medications such as ibuprofen or naproxen can help reduce pain and inflammation.

4. Corticosteroid injections: In some cases, a corticosteroid injection may be given directly into the affected area to help reduce inflammation and pain.

5. Shoulder exercises: Specific

exercises can help improve shoulder strength and flexibility, which can help reduce pain and improve function.

6. Acupuncture: Acupuncture may help reduce pain and improve shoulder function in some patients.

# Peripheral Nerve Stim

Peripheral nerve stimulation (PNS) is a type of pain management therapy that uses electrical impulses to relieve chronic pain. PNS works by delivering small electrical currents to the peripheral nerves, which are the nerves located outside the brain and spinal cord. This stimulation helps to disrupt pain signals sent to the brain and spinal cord, reducing the sensation of pain.

There are several current options for PNS for pain management, including:

1. Traditional PNS: This

involves implanting a small device called a pulse generator beneath the skin near the site of the pain. The device is connected to one or more thin wires called leads, which are inserted near the peripheral nerves. The pulse generator sends electrical impulses to the leads, which in turn stimulate the nerves and help to reduce pain.

2. High-frequency PNS: This involves using a higher frequency of electrical stimulation to disrupt pain signals. This type of PNS is thought to be more effective

at relieving certain types of chronic pain, such as nerve pain and complex regional pain syndrome.

3. Burst PNS: This involves delivering a burst of electrical stimulation to the nerves, rather than a continuous stream of electrical impulses. This can be a more effective way of disrupting pain signals, and may also reduce the amount of energy needed to achieve pain relief.

4. Wireless PNS: This involves using a wireless device to deliver electrical impulses to the nerves. This eliminates

the need for leads, making
the procedure less invasive
and reducing the risk of
complications.

I have had good success with
peripheral nerve stimulation
for patients that have pain
after knee replacements,
chronic inguinal neuralgia
pain, chronic shoulder pain
and low back pain after back
surgery.

# Inguinal Neuralgia

Inguinal neuralgia is a very painful and sometimes difficult pain to treat. It is groin related pain that can occur on it's own but is also sometimes a complication of previous hernia repair. I have seen the most benefit when a multi-modality approach is taken. We generally will start one of the neuropathic pain medications like a Lyrica or Cymbalta to help treat systemically and then will combine this with a targeted peripheral nerve block to the region. For more difficult cases, we will consider peripheral nerve stimulation as described in the past chapter.

## Vitamins and Herbals

There is a specific group of vitamin deficiencies that have been shown to complicate chronic pain and is recommended that all pain patients have lab work performed to rule out a deficiency.  Specifically Vitamin B12 and Vitamin D have been shown to complicate or worsen pain conditions.  Vitamin D deficiency can directly lead to or complicate peripheral neuropathy and other neuropathic pain conditions. Vitamin D deficiency is very common in chronic pain patients and is a common cause of muscle pain or lower extremity cramping.

From a over the counter standpoint I recommend the majority of my patients also consider adding Magnesium as most are deficient. Magnesium is a smooth muscle relaxant and also can help with anxiety.

Other supplements we consider for our patients depending on the underlying problem include:

Glucosamine/Chondroitin combination for arthitic pain.

Turmeric for arthitic pain.

Vitamin B 100 complex and CoQ10 for Headaches.

# CBD and THC

Low-dose THC and CBD oil may be used as part of a comprehensive treatment plan for chronic pain. The exact dosing and formulation will depend on the individual and their specific needs, and it's important to work with a healthcare provider to determine the most appropriate treatment approach.

Here are some current treatment options for chronic pain with low-dose THC and CBD oil:

1. Medical cannabis: In states where medical cannabis is legal, healthcare providers may recommend it as a

treatment option for chronic pain. Medical cannabis typically contains both THC and CBD, and the exact ratio of these cannabinoids will vary depending on the strain and formulation.

2. CBD oil: CBD oil is a non-psychoactive cannabinoid that has been shown to have anti-inflammatory and pain-relieving effects. CBD oil is available in various formulations and dosages, and it's important to work with a healthcare provider to determine the most appropriate product and

dosing for your specific needs.

3. Low-dose THC/CBD oil: Low-dose THC/CBD oil is a product that contains both THC and CBD in specific ratios. This product may be used as part of a comprehensive treatment plan for chronic pain, and it's important to work with a healthcare provider to determine the most appropriate formulation and dosing.

4. Topical CBD products: Topical CBD products, such as creams and lotions, can be

applied directly to the skin to provide localized pain relief. These products may be particularly useful for joint pain and other types of musculoskeletal pain.

In practice, I have found that the greatest benefit of either low dosed THC or CBD products has been with neuropathic pain and with sleep/anxiety.

I generally do not recommend mixing low dose THC or CBD oil products with traditional narcotics.

# Narcotic Management

There is a reason I have waited over 195 pages to finally address narcotic medications and it's place in chronic pain. To be clear narcotics should never be the first line option for chronic pain but in some instances they are a necessary tool that is used. All patients on narcotics need to be warned of the potential pitfalls and dangers of narcotics and should be warned to only take the medication as prescribed. All patients should sign a narcotic medication agreement, undergo ongoing psychological testing and periodic drug screens while on narcotic medication.

Narcotic medications, also known as opioids, are a class of drugs that are commonly used for the management of chronic pain. Opioids work by binding to specific receptors in the brain and spinal cord, which can help to reduce pain perception. There are several different types of opioids available, including natural and synthetic opioids.

Some of the most commonly prescribed opioid medications for chronic pain include:

- Hydrocodone (Vicodin, Norco)

- Oxycodone (OxyContin, Xtampza ER, Percocet)
- Fentanyl Patch
- Morpine (MS Contin)
- Nucynta
- Buprenorphine (Butrans Patch, Suboxone, Belbucca)

While opioids can be effective in reducing pain, they also carry significant risks of dependence, addiction, and overdose. As a result, they are generally reserved for cases of severe or refractory pain and their use is carefully monitored.

The history of opioid use for pain management dates back centuries, with opium being used as a pain reliever in ancient civilizations such as the Greeks and Romans. However, it wasn't until the 19th century that opioids began to be used more widely in Western medicine.

Morphine, which is one of the most potent and effective opioids, was first isolated from opium in the early 1800s. It quickly became a popular pain reliever, particularly during the American Civil War, where it was used to treat soldiers' injuries and alleviate their pain.

Over the years, other opioids have been developed, including codeine, heroin, and synthetic opioids such as fentanyl. In the 20th century, opioids were increasingly prescribed for chronic pain, leading to an epidemic of opioid addiction and overdose deaths.

Today, there is growing recognition of the risks of opioid use, and efforts are being made to limit their use in favor of non-opioid pain management strategies. However, opioids remain an important tool in the management of severe and chronic pain.

Below I will go in further detail of the most interesting and unique narcotic medications that patients in the practice have responded to.

# Nucynta

Nucynta, also known by its generic name tapentadol, is a narcotic pain reliever that is used to treat moderate to severe chronic pain. It works by binding to specific receptors in the brain and spinal cord, which can help to reduce pain perception.

Nucynta is different from other opioid medications in that it also affects the reuptake of norepinephrine, a neurotransmitter that is involved in the body's pain response. This dual mechanism of action means that Nucynta may be more effective at relieving certain types of pain, such as neuropathic pain, than other opioids.

Studies have shown that Nucynta is effective at reducing pain in patients with chronic lower back pain, diabetic neuropathy, and osteoarthritis. Additionally, Nucynta has been shown to have fewer gastrointestinal side effects than other opioids, such as constipation and nausea.

Another benefit of Nucynta is that it has a lower risk of abuse and dependence compared to other opioids. This is because it has a unique chemical structure that makes it more difficult to convert into a form that can be abused.

# Buprenorphine

Buprenorphine is a medication used to treat moderate to severe chronic pain. It is a partial agonist at the mu-opioid receptor, which means that it binds to the same receptors as other opioids but produces a weaker effect.

One of the main benefits of buprenorphine for chronic pain is that it has a lower risk of respiratory depression and overdose compared to other opioid medications. This is because it has a ceiling effect, meaning that after a certain point, further increases in dosage do not produce a greater effect.

In addition to its pain-relieving

properties, buprenorphine is also used to treat opioid addiction. It can help to reduce withdrawal symptoms and cravings, making it easier for people to transition off of stronger opioids like heroin or oxycodone.

Buprenorphine is available in several forms, including sublingual tablets, buccal film (Belbucca), and transdermal patches (Butrans Patch). The sublingual tablets are the most commonly used form for chronic pain management. They are placed under the tongue and allowed to dissolve, which allows the medication to be absorbed into the bloodstream quickly.

# Congrats Pain Warrior!

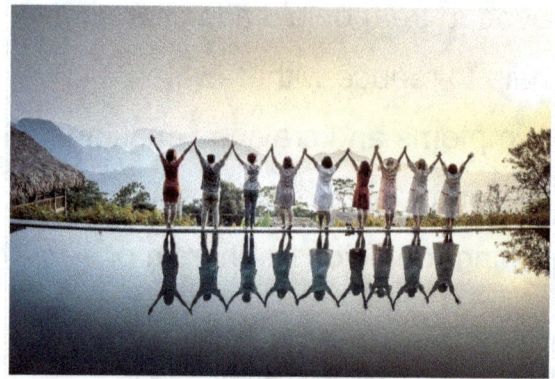

I want to send a congratulations to anyone who took the time to make it through my 204 page ultimate guide to pain management! I hope you have found some useful information and have come to realize that their is hope for treating your chronic pain.  I truly believe that every patient in pain can find a decreased level of pain and improved level of function. As this book details, it takes you being an active participant in your treatment. Find yourself a local multidisciplinary team to help you on your journey. I hope my insights from my past 23 years of practice have given you some actionable information to discuss with your local healthcare providers. For taking on this journey to be an active participant you are no longer merely a patient instead you are a warrior, a Pain Warrior. You will continue to battle and not give in to the pain. I am confident you will find peace and success along your journey!

## About the Author

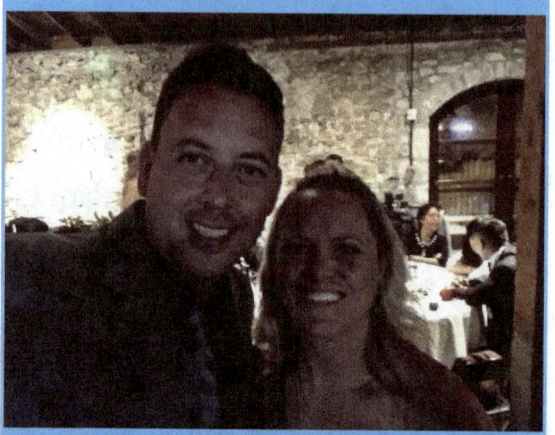

Matthew Dovie has been the head APP at Lanier Interventional Pain Center in Gainesville, GA for the past 23 years. You can find out more about the practice at lanierpain.com

www.ingramcontent.com/pod-product-compliance
Lightning Source LLC
Chambersburg PA
CBHW070539220526
45467CB00003B/999